Lyme Disease: Natural Treatment Solutions to Heal Yourself

Cure your Lyme disease symptoms in just a few days with our safe and natural treatment solution!

Written By: Alyson Rodgers

Published by:

Alyson Rodgers and Random Technologies

4409 HOFFNER AVENUE, SUITE 347

Belle Isle, FL 32812

Disclaimer

This book is intended as a reference material, not as a medical manual to replace the advice of your physician or to substitute for any treatment prescribed by your physician.

If you are ill or suspect that you have a medical problem, we strongly encourage you to consult your medical, health, or other competent professional before adopting any of the suggestions in this book or drawing inferences from it. If you are taking prescription medication, you should never change your diet (for better or worse) without consulting your physician, as any dietary change may affect the metabolism of that prescription drug.

This book and the author's opinions are solely for informational and educational purposes.

The author specifically disclaims all responsibility for any liability, loss, or risk, personal or otherwise which is incurred as a consequence, directly or indirectly, of the use and application of any of the contents of this book. Individual results may vary.

Table of Contents

Welcome

The most common tick-borne disease in the United States was originally named after a town in Connecticut where a group of children experienced arthritis like symptoms. With over 15,000 new cases reported each year, Lyme disease is becoming more widespread across the United States, with more and more individuals experiencing symptoms of their own.

Despite the availability of a number of treatments for the disease that is spread by the common deer tick, experts believe that improvements can be made in the area.

This report will discuss a natural remedy that offers a more holistic approach to the treatment of Lyme disease that aids and abets the role of prescribed antibiotics and medicines. The new approach looks to target both the root cause and the symptoms and provides a more complete approach to health and wellbeing in the context of Lyme disease. The report will outline the improvements that can be made in the treatment of Lyme disease when using the unique and natural approach, before the conclusion will sum up the most important points to take from the research and associated commentary.

Number Of Cases

Lyme disease is arguably the fastest-growing epidemic in the world.

The Center for Disease Control (CDC) in Atlanta, Georgia, U.S.A. suggests that "there is considerable under-reporting" of Lyme disease, and maintains that the actual infection rate may be 1.8 million, 10 times higher than the 180,000 cases currently reported. Nick Harris, Ph.D., Director of the International Lyme and Associated Diseases Society (ILADS), explains that "Lyme is grossly under-reported. In the U.S., we probably have about 200,000 cases per year."

In support of that statement, Dan Kinderleher, M.D., an expert on Lyme disease, stated on the Today Show on June 10, 2002 that the number of cases may be 100 times higher (18 million in the United States alone) than reported by the CDC.

Jo Anne Whitaker, M.D., has developed a "Rapid Identification of Borrelia burgdorferi" and has over 2900 positive specimens for Bb from forty-six (46) states, including Alaska and Hawaii. In addition, Dr. Whitaker has had positive specimens from Canada, Brazil, Denmark, Scotland, The Netherlands, Ireland, England, France, Spain, Germany, Switzerland, and the Canary Islands.

Considering vector, congenital and sexual transfer, Dr. Harvey and Dr. Salvato estimate that 15.5% of the global population, nearly 1 billion people, could be infected with Bb. Lee Cowden, M.D., states that there are very few symptoms where one should not consider Lyme, especially given that a quarter of the U.S. population may be affected. It is estimated that Lyme disease may be a contributing factor in more than 50% of chronically ill people.

This report aims to empower readers with the ability to confront the detrimental effects of the disease by controlling medication, diet and preventative techniques associated with Lyme disease. While the report focuses on the effects of Lyme disease specifically, it also provides broader principles of health and wellness, which will increase the reader's awareness of holistic therapies and pain relief.

In doing so, the report will touch on subjects that may be beyond the comprehension of the average reader. Therefore, In addition to broadening the readers own knowledge of Lyme disease, the collection of resources gathered might prove helpful to the medical professional entrusted to abate the illness. Accordingly, it is important to consult a health professional in the treatment of the disease, and this report is provided as a guide only, and is not a substitute for qualified medical advice.

Report Overview

The report that follows is a collection of important information about the disease and the best ways in which to fight it. Please take the time to read through the whole document. This gives you the best opportunity to reduce your pain and suffering and to hasten your return to full health.   The report contains the following sections:

Chapter 1: Overview of Lyme Disease. Learn what it is, what causes it, who's at risk, how it is diagnosed, what are the signs and symptoms, and typical complications.

Chapter 2: Lyme Disease Remedies. Learn about traditional-medication remedies, diet remedies, and alternative-treatment remedies that you can easily provide for yourself in your own home.

Chapter 3: Living With Lyme Disease. Discover what you can do as a Lyme disease sufferer to manage your episodes, their pain, and frequency. Learn how to mitigate the effects of Lyme disease and to limit and/or eliminate chronic damage caused by it. Learn how to diagnose, prevent, and treat Lyme disease in your family's pets.

Chapter 4: Concluding Thoughts about You, Your Health, and Lyme Disease. Consider your role in your overall health and contemplate what opportunities a pain-free life would make available to you.

Bonus Materials: Check out the best the Web has to offer in Lyme disease resources.

What is Lyme Disease?

Chapter one looks at the origin of Lyme disease and how it affects the population. With particular emphasis on what causes the disease and which demographic is the most susceptible, the following passages will heighten your knowledge of the subject and provide the catalyst for taking charge of your health.

What Is It?

Lyme disease (LD) is a bacterial infection caused by Borrelia burgdorferi, a type of bacterium called a spirochete that is carried by the common black-legged, or deer, tick. Infected ticks transmit the spirochete to the humans and animals it bites. If left untreated, the bacterium will travel through the host body's bloodstream and situate itself within a variety of body tissues. The results are many and varied, including such things as rashes, flu-like symptoms, and aching joints that mimic arthritis.

Without treatment, Lyme disease can cause serious, long-term health problems, but Lyme disease can often be treated with antibiotics.

How Does An Individual Get Lyme Disease?

Quite simply, in order for an individual to contract the disease, a tick carrying the above bacteria must bite them.

Only two species of ticks, both belonging to the "Ixode" genus, are carriers: Deer Ticks (Ixodes scapularis), and Black-Legged Ticks (Ixode pacificus). Ixode ticks are found mainly on deer, although field mice, rabbits, sheep, and cattle may also pick them up.

After a tick has become infected, it can infect any organism it bites. However, even after being bitten by a carrying tick, an individual may not develop the disease. Quite fortunately, the tick needs to remain attached to its host body for thirty six hours before the bacteria will infect the bloodstream and materialize into Lyme disease.

Where Is Lyme Disease Found?

Recent statistics show that cases of Lyme disease have been reported in nearly every U.S. state as well as within Europe and Asia. Interestingly the majority of reported cases are centralized to the following regions:

1. Northern California

2. Eastern Coastal states such as Connecticut, Delaware, Maryland, New Jersey, New York, and Rhode Island

3. Northern Central states such as Wisconsin

What Are The Most Common Symptoms of Lyme Disease?

The symptoms associated with Lyme disease can vary dramatically and ultimately depend on which body tissue the disease primarily resides in. In addition to sharing symptoms with a host of other more common diseases and conditions, at times this can pose difficulties in assessing the impact of Lyme disease and the correct treatment plan, however the most common symptoms include:

- Intense fatigue
- Diminished or absent reflexes
- Brain fog
- Insomnia or excessive sleep
- Memory loss (short & long term)
- Joint pain/swelling/stiffness
- Poor coordination/ataxia

- Difficulty reading
- Slow or slurred speech
- Unexplained chills & fevers
- Rash
- Sudden abrupt mood swings
- Continual infections
- Poor concentration
- Decreased ability to spell correctly
- Unusual depression
- Tremors
- Disorientation
- Burning/stabbing pain
- Facial paralysis (Bell's Palsy)
- GI distress/abdominal pain
- Poor word retrieval/Aphasia
- Shortness of breath
- Anxiety
- Heart palpitations/chest pain
- Weight changes (loss or gain)
- Difficulty swallowing
- Sore throat
- Swollen glands
- Nausea/vomiting
- Anorexia
- Cough
- Vasculitis
- Muscle pain or cramps
- Loss of muscle tone
- Changes in taste or smell
- Twitching of muscles (face or other)
- Obsessive-Compulsive symptoms
- Panic attacks
- Changes in cerebral blood flow/brain waves

- Peripheral neuropathy/tingling/numbness
- Number reversal
- Lightheadedness
- Headaches/Migraines
- Light Sensitivity
- Menstrual irregularities
- Change in hearing/buzzing/tinnitus
- Trigeminal neuralgia (TMJ)
- Unexplained hair loss
- Dilated cardiomyopathy
- Visual disturbance
- Loss of temperature control

Potentially the most obvious and visible indication of infection is the red rash known as erythema migraines. Not to be confused with the original bite mark, the rash measures approximately two inches and takes the impression of an inflamed red circle. Although not painful, nor itchy, the rash may feel warm to touch and usually develops within thirty days of being bitten.

If the rash is left undetected or ignored, it can spread to other parts of the body. In extreme cases this can spread rapidly and within days, but in other cases it can take weeks to develop. Complications can develop which can cause Bell's palsy, intense headaches and stiffness due to meningitis, heart palpitations and dizziness and shooting pains. Failing to detect or treat the area results in arthritis symptoms with intense joint pain and swelling, most often in the knees, in 60% of instances, and for low number of cases, the disease can mean chronic neurological issues, including numbness in the hands or feet and short term memory loss.

Alarmingly, individuals who seek treatment may still experience some of the ongoing symptoms listed above that can cause discomfort for months in minor cases to years in extreme situations.

How Is Lyme Disease Diagnosed?

Not every test currently designed to detect Lyme disease is 100% accurate, thus making the detection of the disease difficult. This is largely due to the fact that the symptoms associated with Lyme disease mimic those of other diseases and conditions. More often than not a correct diagnosis depends on the assessment of whether the individual has come into contact with an infected tick, or the possibility that they have.

Serologic testing is the main option to assist medical professionals in identifying the disease, but a more modern approach of "PCR" testing is being developed to objectively determine the presence of the bacteria in tissue, blood and body fluids. This should see improvements in the area and go some way in diminishing the psychological impact of uncertainty amongst potentially infected individuals.

Who Is at Risk of Lyme Disease?

As the description above stipulates, no one demographic is at more risk of contracting Lyme disease. Because the infection is reliant on a single bite, the chances of contracting the disease are increased in those that spend time in areas of trees, bush and scrub. The same can be said for

Nevertheless, it's important to remain vigilant especially for those living in the four most susceptible regions listed above. For those that are anxious about the possibility of infection or simply want more information on their susceptibility to the disease, our strong recommendation is that you contact a health professional.

Lyme disease's futile nature outlines the importance of early detection, before it consumes the individual's mind and body.

Next, we'll look at the Lyme disease is commonly treated and we'll introduce our unique home remedy solution, which will dramatically improve the management of symptoms and likelihood of a full recovery.

Lyme Disease Solutions

After reading the first chapter you're probably a little confused about how such a troublesome disease has flown under the radar of publicity and awareness. When the complicated testing procedures are combined with the commonplace symptoms it is often difficult to comprehend how the disease can be treated effectively. The good news is, that many of the treatments available enjoy considerable success in treating the symptoms and easing the pain. More so, recent research around the holistic approach suggests a more natural approach can improve victims overall health.

With effective treatment, sufferers can usually:

- Rid themselves of the infection;

- Alleviate the pain associated with the disease; and

- Prevent future symptoms.

With early detection, the chances of treating Lyme disease improve to the point where treatment can cure each and every aspect of the disease. As previously alluded to, treatment, can mean the medicine prescribed by your health professional and the home remedies and nutritional changes you can make to take control over the disease. Traditional medicines have their place in dealing with Lyme disease, but so too, does holistic therapy and supplementary treatment that targets over wellbeing rather than the isolation of Lyme disease.

The Medical Industry Approach

Following a prescribed regimen of oral antibiotics over a period of a few weeks can cure most cases of Lyme disease. Antibiotics commonly used for oral treatment include doxycycline, amoxicillin, or cefuroxime axetil. Only in rare cases, usually involving neurological or cardiac complications, will patients require intravenous treatment with drugs such as ceftriaxone or penicillin. The pharmaceutical approach uses the following antibiotics and approaches:

Tetracycline
Tetracyclines including doxycycline are the first choice for treating Lyme disease. However, tetracyclines can cause a wide range of side effects, including gastric irritation, nausea, vomiting, diarrhea, kidney toxicity, liver toxicity, and alterations in blood coagulation. Permanent staining of the teeth may also result if tetracyclines are given to young children, a consequence also observed in children whose mothers took tetracycline during pregnancy. Like all broad spectrum antibiotics, tetracycline kills 'good' as well as 'bad' bacteria, leaving the user with lower immunity levels and facing the risk of Candida yeast overgrowth in the mouth, vagina, and bowel. Consequently, the good intestinal bacteria should be replaced with probiotic supplementation after a course of antibiotics.

A further option in the fight against Lyme disease is the use of Cephalosporins (ceftriaxone). In contrast to the use of Tetracyclines, these are not the first option in treatment plans because of their relative difficulty to administer. I.e. they can only be given intravenously or by intramuscular injection, rather than orally. They are used mainly where individuals show negative reactions to the other options or where others haven't had the desired effect. Disappointingly, they are expensive and are often overlooked for that reason. As with all medicines they can give off side effects ranging from gall bladder inflammation to intestinal overgrowth of Candida yeast.

Macrolides (erythromycin)
Marcolides tend to do more to prevent the harmful bacteria from reproducing rather than attacking the root cause of the disease. In the treatment of Lyme disease, Marcolides are prescribed in high doses but have only brought moderate success in studies conducted to assess their performance. In some cases the intake of this option can cause gastrointestinal distress and yeast overgrowth, making them unsuitable for long-term use.

Vaccination
Upon the successful completion of animal vaccination over a course of years, scientists have been developing a human vaccine that looks to stimulate anti-Borrelia production and therefore reduce the risks of contracting Lyme disease. Despite controversy and discontent in some circles, the vaccination program looks set to continue through the FDA.

Length of Treatment
Those infected with the disease that accept treatment early, are expected to make a hasty and complete recovery. The length of treatment can however be extended if diagnosis is only given when the disease is in the latter stages. In those cases, it is recommended that individuals take a second course of treatment but also exhibit extreme care due to the risks associated with long-term antibiotic treatments and potential health complications.

Treatment and Pregnancy

Pregnancy has no great influence on the treatment of Lyme disease. Studies have concluded that unless the antibiotics prescribed pose a danger to the unborn child, then there should be no change in the treatment plan from that of an otherwise healthy adult. As always however, it's important to exercise caution and speak to a health professional if you're in this position.

Natural Treatment Solutions

As a general disclaimer to the following information, those who are or suspect they have been exposed to Lyme disease should in the first instance consult a medical professional to determine the best course of action in testing and treating for the disease. Medical professionals are the best equipped to alleviate pain and alleviate the affect the disease can have on the human body.

Using the treatments and antibiotics described above, medical professionals succeed in treating the disease because of the aggressive nature of the drugs and the aggressive impact it has on the bloodstream. The flipside of such a treatment is that the body struggles to maintain the level of defense against other complications and side effects. This means any treatment plan can have detrimental effects on the body, the height of which can be fatal.

Because of this, and because of the subtitles in individual cases of Lyme disease, we recommend alternative treatments to supplement the sometime harsh effects of traditional plans. The remedies that we suggest have shown to address the root cause of the disease by cleansing the body of harmful toxins and bacteria. As the sub-title of the report stipulates, the benefits of the alternative treatments can be seen in less than seventy two hours. Here's how:

The 3 Day Solution: The Power of Salt and Vitamin C

The remedy is based on the research of the Nobel Prize-winning scientist Linus Pauling and other leading edge theorists. It cunningly uses two common household items (salt and vitamin C) and combines them into a holistic approach that attacks the cause of the disease. Surprising, the two household items that have been credited with revolutionizing the holistic treatment of Lyme disease are also ones that are often associated with moderation.

Despite the warnings placed over the consumption of salt, research suggests we're actually consuming much less than we did historically. Ironically, this coincides with the increase in know and reported cases of Lyme disease, making the logic behind using it in the seventy two hour remedy to be sound. To add to that, vitamin c can also play a significant role in assisting affected Lyme carriers. The U.S. Recommended Daily Allowance of Vitamin C is a mere 60 milligrams per day, but researchers like Pauling are suggesting 18,000 milligrams per day would result in profound benefits for preventive health. This all makes for exciting times in the advancement of Lyme disease treatment.

The science behind the unique combination shows a systematic eradication of the bacteria associated with Lyme disease. But, it's even more effective than that. Recent research is showing the possibility of other pathogens being associated with Lyme disease, and the seventy two hour remedy painlessly rids the body of bacteria, mites and worms.

Dose
- 12-one gram tablets of salt. One brand of salt pill is CMC (Consolidated Midland Corporation), NDC#0223-1760-01, ordered through a pharmacy (no prescription required)

- 12-1,000 mg tablets of Vitamin C
- Water

The home remedy requires the taking the above dose every hour throughout the day with food and in conjunction with a considerable amount of water. Trials of the home remedy show that the most effective results occur when the dose is gradually increased, rather than immediate and large quantities.

An example of a gradual-dose protocol would begin with a dose of 1 gram each of salt and Vitamin C at 10 am and again at 2 PM. If you experience fatigue or have a mild feeling of malaise, omit a 6 PM dose. Instead, drink plenty of water through the rest of the day and evening. Maintain a schedule of just 2 doses per day until there is no reaction (which may take 1 or 2 days), then move on to 3 doses per day with the addition of a dose at 6 PM.

All in all, this helps the body acclimatize to the remedy, and is proven to deliver optimum results in the treatment of Lyme disease. Rather than reducing the body's good bacteria, this approach strengthens the body's defensive mechanisms and cleanses the body of toxins harmful to everyday life not just harmful in treating Lyme disease.

If after 72 hours you do not feel better, repeat the remedy once every 3-5 days until you notice the benefits.

Why does it work?
The system is so effective because of the impact the dose has on our white blood cells. White blood cells play an important role in defending the body and attacking so called bad bacteria. One class of white blood cells in particular has areas where they store an enzyme that uses an acid, along with hydrogen peroxide, to produce an oxygen particle (electron) that kills invading microbes. In other words, it creates and uses a free radical molecule to protect itself.

Another area of storage in these same white blood cells contains different types of proteins (polypeptides), one of which is called

cathelicidin. A segment of this protein is a potential bacteria killer (bacteriacide) that increases the "permeability" of the bacteria's cell membrane which ultimately kills them.

One enzyme, called "elastase" a series of short protein peptides, are able to be assembled into larger ones (dubbed "LL-37") that are able to increase the "permeability" of the bacteria's cell membrane.

These two enzymes work together when they meet an offending bacterium. The elastase uses some of the cathelicidins to pull out a protein molecule from the surface membrane of bacteria. This causes an opening or "pore" to form in the membrane itself. This allows vital potassium ions needed by the microorganism to escape from within its internal walls (the Borrelia's "cytoplasm") and out through the "pore". This damages the bacteria internally, resulting in swelling and eventually ruptures the microorganism.

Increasing the salt in the body fluids surrounding the Borrelia bacteria contributes to the killing effect by allowing sodium ions to enter the bacteria through the "pore" created by the anti-microbial peptides. The increased level of sodium in the bacteria, combined with the loss of needed potassium, enhances the killing effect further.

Vitamin C is known to increase the number and activity of white blood cells. People infected with Lyme disease often have lower white blood cell counts due to the ongoing infection. So, in addition to the known anti-microbial "osmotic pressure effect" of salt, it appears the Vitamin C may increase the number and activity of the white blood cells needed, and then the increased salt levels in the intra cellular fluid "arms" them with Borrelia-killing enzymes and peptides.

Common Side Effects

As with any treatment plan, the seventy two hour natural method can have some side effects on the hosts body. Most of those infected with Lyme disease will accept some side effects, mainly due to the amazing results seen in such a short space of time after beginning the plan. It is important to note that the side effects can include diarrhea (which is a sign that the body is beginning to flush out the toxins associated with Lyme), fever, chills, muscle pain, headaches, skin lesions, nausea, and soreness of the throat.

Facts about Salt

Much has been written in recent years about "too much salt" being "bad for you". Studies were conducted which suggested higher salt intake increased incidence of high-blood pressure. However, other researchers subsequently called the studies into question, particularly how these studies were conducted.

However, the type of salt central to these studies was typical westernized, refined or processed "table salt". This has been found, and has been known for years in alternative health circles, to be extremely detrimental to human health. Not all salt is created equal. They may all taste salty but they are different in action and function.

What Exactly is Refined or Processed Table Salt?

Beginning in 1923, processors began kiln-drying salt at temperatures above 400 degrees. This changed the chemical structure of salt. During the refining process, 82 out of 84 mineral elements are removed. Normally, only 7% of all the sea salt processed is used for human consumption. The majority of the sea salt is sold for industrial use, and has great commercial value. It is used in the silver mining process. Boron is extracted to make anti-knock gasoline additives and chemical fertilizers. Magnesium is sold to makers of metal alloys and for explosives. Other chemicals are removed from salt to make plastics. Then, after taking all of the natural, but salable, mineral elements out of the salt, chemicals are added to bleach it whiter and to prevent water absorption while the salt is in the box.

Table salt is basically an inorganic sodium compound to which additives have been added such as aluminum hydroxide, silica aluminate, sodium ferrocyanide, Tri-calcium phosphate, stearic acid and others. The aluminum additives leave a bitter taste so the manufacturers add dextrose, a refined sugar, which disrupts the body's equilibrium. Plus, aluminum has been implicated in Alzheimer's disease.

This inorganic, processed compound is actually toxic to the body and causes it to retain fluid in an effort to keep this toxin in suspension. The same chemicals added to salt to prevent water absorption in the box also prevent it from being properly absorbed in your body.

This is why we hear that salt's bad for you. Refined salt is bad for you. It can be deposited in the joints of your bones, and cause arthritis. Some of it can be deposited in the walls of your arteries and veins, lymph system ducts, sexual organs, urinary tract, or glandular system. It can cause the body to retain water which can cause swelling, bloating, edema, and cellulite. This will only occur with long term use.

People today are starving for minerals that have been removed from both the soil and the salt. What do doctors prescribe to help regulate manic-depressive individuals? Lithium, a trace mineral in sea salt that is removed from table salt. Iodized salt became commonly available in the 1930s only after a large percentage of the population developed goiter in response to iodine deficiency. These are the body's responses to only two instances of mineral deficiency. It's reasonable to ask what damage is being done due to the lack of the other 80 minerals normally available to us through salt consumption.

Rock salt or sea salt is loaded with minerals. This was the type of salt with which Roman soldiers were paid, thus the word salary. They ate 25 grams per day just as early American settlers ate 20 grams per day. We recommend eating only sea salt and avoiding processed table salt for regular dietary use. Avoid eating processed foods, restaurant foods, and other prepared foods that use table salt. RealSalt, Celtic Sea Salt, or any naturally evaporated sea or rock salt are brands worth considering for everyday use. As a bonus, natural sea salt is not only extremely beneficial and rich in minerals, it has a delicious, gourmet taste, by itself and on any food.

Why is table salt recommended in the form of CMC (Consolidated Midland Corporation) NDC#0223-1760-01?

This salt tablet is used for the protocol due to its dose (1000 mg), ease of use and the fact that sea salt minerals may create issues with effectiveness of the cure. This brand has been used successfully so why change it. Use of CMC salt will create no ill effects for the length of time needed to eradicate your Lyme disease. You can change over to sea salt after the protocol has done its job in ridding you of the infection. After all, lack of salt in the diet created the crack in our immunity armor. By maintaining the levels of salt in the system after the protocol has been finished, you can ensure that any residual pockets of bacteria can't multiply and will be eventually eradicated.

How Supplements Can Help

One of the most obvious but often overlooked measures an individual can take to increase their chances of a speedy Lyme disease recovery is to maintain a balanced and healthy diet, consisting of the optimum levels of vitamins, nutrients and minerals. Diets can be difficult to maintain in the face of fast paced lifestyles and work and family pressures, but allowing this to serve as an excuse in the fight to counteract Lyme disease is concerning. As such an easy aspect of your life and treatment plant to control, a balanced diet boosts the immune system and fuels the body in its fight against Lyme disease.

Cats Claw

There are over 300 conditions connected to Lyme disease according to the article Hidden Plague, Forget About SARS by Dr. Whitaker. Lyme disease is spreading steadily, and some experts say it can elude the standard cure of antibiotic use. Reported in an article in the June 16, 2003 issue of People Magazine, one patient suffering from Lyme disease was misdiagnosed with Lou Gehrig's disease (ALS), an incurable disease that is fatal within 5 years of onset. Dr. Whitaker states that nearly every patient she has tested who is suffering from Parkinson's disease has tested positive for Bb, the bacterium indicating Lyme disease.

Samento is a form of Cat's Claw from the Peruvian jungle that is superior to typical forms. The beneficial effects of most Cat's Claw preparations are blunted by the presence of TOA (tetracyclic oxindole alkaloids), which inhibit the real active agents, called POA (pentacyclic oxindole alkaloids). The latter, more favorable compounds are known to modulate and up-regulate the immune system. Many commercially available Cat's Claw preparations contain up to 80% TOA. As little as 1% TOA can reduce POA effectiveness up to 80%. In addition, the specific species of TOA-free cat's claw contains considerable quantities of quinovic acid glycosides. These compounds are what the latest generation of quinolone antibiotics (such as Cipro) are based on. The natural compounds provide safe and significant direct antimicrobial effects on Lyme disease.

Professor Luis Romero, M.D., Ph.D., reports three patients that had been diagnosed with Parkinson's disease years ago to be 99%

reversed using Pentacyclic Alkaloid Chemotype Uncaria tomentosa. (TOA-Free Cat's Claw - Prima Unã De Gato) Pentacyclic Alkaloid Chemotype Uncaria tomentosa has been available to the public in Bulgaria, where a high incidence of Lyme disease exists, since January 2001. Within 2 months, it became the most widely sold natural medicine in that country.

Dr. Atanas Tzonkov, director of Bulgaria's largest private medical clinic, has treated thousands of patients with Pentacyclic Alkaloid Chemotype Uncaria tomentosa (Cats Claw). He reports that it has been used successfully to treat over 100 different conditions. A possible theory is that most of these conditions were actually misdiagnosed Lyme disease or that Lyme disease was a component of the illnesses afflicting those patients.

Treatment with TOA-free cat's claw isn't an instant cure-all. It can take a long treatment process because of the variety of forms of Bb, the long length of time it can exist in the body in the CWD form, and because it can hide out inside cells. It is when they emerge that they are susceptible to white cell attack and elimination. The mature spirochete form is sensitive to attack by antibiotics or the immune system, as well as the improved Cat's Claw. The organism can lie dormant for months or years after infection. In fact, a 1998 Swiss study showed that only 12.5 percent of Bb positive patients have symptoms. Three companies currently market the improved Cat's Claw:

- Allergy Research Group/Nutricology, can be reached at 800-545-9960 or www.nutricology.com. Ask for Prima Una de Gato.

- Nutramedix's product is called Samento Plus, and is available by calling 561-745-2917 or on the web at: www.nutramedix.com.

- Farmacopia also carries the product. You can contact them at 800-896-1484 or on the web at: www.farmacopia.net

Multivitamins

A high quality multi-vitamin provides further ammunition to boost immunity and energy. Most standard multi-vitamins on the market are suitable to supplement the body's efforts against Lyme disease.

Vitamin A

Vitamin A deficiency can slow the potential for the body to fight infection and alleviate pain and a top up of Vitamin A can only assist in the fight for optimum health. Early research on the topic and from field studies in animals show that increased Vitamin A levels help alleviate arthritic pain and inflammation. Once again, this is an easy and relatively risk free addition to any treatment plan that can help individuals struggling with the symptoms of Lyme disease.

Lactobacillus acidophilus and bifidobacteria

Long courses of antibiotics have shown to have detrimental effects on bodies already locked in ongoing battles with the illness and the disease. That is why the consumption of Probiotics tablets are strongly recommended to \ help minimize the risk of bad bacteria multiplying and causing havoc. Focusing mainly on the stomach, and in more detail, the acidity of the stomach, probiotics contain freeze-dried bacteria or powders that contain live cultures.

One such variety of potent probiotics is HSO (Homeostatic Soil Organisms), Colostrum is also a good supplement for boosting overall immune function.

Omega 3 Essential Fatty Acids

As mentioned in a host of articles, studies and research on diets and healthy lifestyles, oils such as fish oil, flaxseed oil and omega 3's are also advised to increase the consumption of the body's essential fatty acids. These oils, which restore the body to its natural level (which can only be achieved with food or capsules), help with inflammation and joint pain.

Antioxidant Nutrients

Because Lyme disease can have such a significant impact on the body tissue throughout the human body, it is essential to control inflammation and take every available measure to boost an immune system. A proper recipe of supplements should include taking vitamins A, C, E, beta-carotene, selenium, coenzyme Q10, and lipoic acid on a regular basis. Antioxidants neutralize free radicals, and with the proper program and professional advice can drastically assist the body in its fight against the nasty tick infection.

Though the list of antioxidants may seem overwhelming they differ in suggested dosage, schedules, cautionary rules, etc. an established routine will soon make the program more comfortable and easier to administer (see below):

- Bromelain acts much like an NSAID. Suggested dose: 2 x 500 mg daily.

- MSM is a methyl donor and is the transport molecule for elemental sulfur or assimilable source of essential sulfur which is required for proper assimilation of the alpha amino acids methionine and cysteine. In addition, the peptide hormone, insulin requires sulfur in its molecular structure. Numerous other proteins, catalysts, and enzymes incorporate sulfur into their molecular framework. Proteins are essential for proper cellular metabolism and soft tissue synthesis. Proper protein synthesis can only be achieved with MSM monomers which maintain the correct molecular framework for soft and connective tissue throughout the human body. Daily dosages of 2,000 to 4,000 mg are recommended.

- Co-Q10 helps the body to increase stamina, fight infections more aggressively, and improve heart function. CoQ10's key role is in producing adenosine triphosphate (ATP), needed for energy production in every cell of the body. Secondary to that, CoQ10 functions as a powerful antioxidant. Suggested dose: 200-300 mg daily.

- DMSO (dimethylsulfoxide) has been shown to relieve joint pain from inflammation and is very effective in relieving pain and swelling caused by inflammation. Suggested doses vary. Check with your doctor for your correct dosage.

- L-glutamine acts much like an antacid and can help inflammation and associated pain. Suggested dose: 4 x 500 mg daily on an empty stomach.

- L-glycine acts much like an antacid and can help inflammation and associated pain. Suggested dose: 4 x 500 mg daily on an empty stomach.

- Shark cartilage has actually been found helpful in eliminating much of the pain associated with Lyme disease. Suggested dose: Take 3-6 capsules daily until pain subsides.

- Vitamin C is the wonder vitamin. Because it lowers uric acid levels, vitamin C can be used for maintenance as well as during an acute Lyme disease attack. Suggested doses: During intense joint pain, 1,000 mg per hour until you reach bowel tolerance indicated by diarrhea. For maintenance, 500-3,000 mg daily.

Herbal Solutions

Continuing the theme of simple measures individuals can take in a holistic sense to improve the chances against Lyme disease is the use of common garden herbs. Nutritionists often suggest the addition of herbs to meals and although they do add to the taste of dishes, the benefits also run through to the body of the recipient. The following herbal pills and extracts help the immune system immensely:

- Dried extracts-which include capsules, powders, and/or teas);

- Glycerites (glycerine extracts); and

- Tinctures (alcohol-based extracts).

Reishi Mushroom

Little known mushroom variety, the Reishi, is known as the mushroom of immortality in China, and for good reason. Reishi is a natural anti-viral agent that protects the blood and liver functions and has been the subject of a host of studies in patients undergoing chemotherapy. Results seem to indicate that most patients who participated in the trials handled their chemotherapy better with the aid of Reishi and enjoyed normal levels of white blood cells, despite the treatments often reducing such counts.

Boswellia

We've discussed at length how commonly found supplements can aid the fight against Lyme disease. These measures traditionally support medicinal treatment options and promote a better overall health foundation. The measures are a simple and cost effective addition to a diet, making the use of them in the battle to better health understandable.

However, some holistic medicines are less well known, but provide similar benefits to the supplements already listed. The first of which is a gummy resin native to India called, Boswellia serrate. Those familiar with holistic medicine will know Boswelia for its contribution to improving symptoms of arthritis, dysentery, liver diseases, obesity, neurological disorders, ringworm, boils, and more. Reports tend to suggest that the super herb has tremendous success in reducing inflammation, without breaking down the joint cartilage like traditional steroid based solutions tend to. Active ingredients in the herb called "Boswellic acids" block the production of potent, tissue-damaging chemicals called "leukotriene's" that are key players in the inflammatory response, rein in the complement system, and check the infiltration of white blood cells into tissues.

Turmeric
Much like Boswelia above, Turmeric works to reduce inflammation without the debilitating muscle and joint effects described earlier. The presence of free-radical fighting abilities have shown (in animal and human studies) that Turmeric has plenty to offer us in terms of antioxidant and anti-inflammatory properties. Containing curcumin, Turmeric lends support to the traditional use of turmeric in arthritis and inflammation-related conditions by inhibiting the enzymes which serve as the catalysts for inflammation.

In a positive endorsement for its potential use to treat Lyme disease, Turmeric (and Curcumin) helped individuals with rheumatoid arthritis in clinical trials. While trials have not been conducted specifically for Lyme disease, the signs point to some arthritic improvements in subjects, and it is therefore probably worth trying in the management of pain connected with Lyme disease.

Grapefruit Seed Extract
Grapefruit seed extract provides yet another option for the holistic treatment of the increasingly common Lyme disease. It is listed as a broad-spectrum antimicrobial substance and appears to break down the cell membranes of bacteria that invade the body, causing them to

die.

In balance with its fighting qualities, grapefruit seed extract also promotes the growth of friendly flora and disease-fighting organisms in the stomach. By controlling yeast overgrowth, test-tube studies suggest grapefruit seed extract also preserves the structural integrity of stomach wall tissue. In one particular human study, an improvement in constipation, gas, abdominal distress, and night rest were noticed after four weeks of therapy with grapefruit seed extract. Most clinicians now agree on the importance of maintaining the correct balance of gut organisms in health and disease. (17, 18)

Oregano Oil
Increasingly popular as an anti-bacterial and anti-fungal agent, Oregano oil, could have an impact on Lyme disease as well. Although there exists no proven data to support this assumption, the consensus is that infection levels could diminish if supplemented correctly in the right conditions. In a recently published clinical trial, Oil of Oregano was given orally to 14 adults whose stools tested positive for intestinal parasites. After six weeks of supplementation with 600mg emulsified Oil of Oregano daily, infection levels dropped sharply, and in some cases disappeared altogether. Gastrointestinal symptoms improved in 7 of the 11 patients. (19)

Oregano also has reported antioxidant activity. The ingredients responsible for this include flavonoids (rosmarinic acid) and vitamin E. Rosmarinic acid is yet another anti-inflammatory herbal ingredient. Also found in rosemary and basil, rosmarinic acid works to check the various enzymes discussed earlier that set the inflammatory process in motion. Going one step further, rosmarinic acid increases the production a beneficial type of prostaglandin that discourages inflammation. This coupled with its supportive influence on the immune system makes Oregano a potentially useful herb in natural therapy for cancer, inflammation, immune-related problems, and Lyme disease. (20-26)

If Oregano oil sounds like a suitable option for you, but you're on other courses of antibiotics, it's important to consult your medical practitioner as to the suitability of taking it. The reason being, oregano oil in rare cases can heighten the impact of traditional medicine and may take you over the prescribed dose of your recommended treatment.

Olive Leaf
In a similar manner to the benefits prescribed by a good quality olive oil, the leaf of the olive tree is said to be an effective ally against a wide variety of infectious microorganisms, including Salmonella typhi, Vibrio parahaemolyticus, and Staphylococcus aureus (including penicillin-resistant strains); and Klebsiella pneumonia and Escherichia coli, causal agents of intestinal or respiratory tract infections in man (28). In lab studies, oleuropein shows the ability to stimulate immune cells in the body called "macrophages which function as garbage collectors to remove organisms and other foreign substances" (30).

In summary, this equates to a strong possibility that olive leaf can against viral infection, and subsequently, Lyme disease.

Homeopathic Solutions

By definition homeopathic treatments, are alternatives. However that is not to say they are any less effective than traditional medicines and treatments. In fact, homeopathic remedies are full of potency when fighting the symptoms of Lyme disease based on the principle of treating like with like. If you take a nosode (a remedy created from the bacterium that causes Lyme disease in the first place), called borrelia burgdorferi, in a 30c potency three times per day, you can actually halt the advance of the disease in its earliest stages.

Homeopaths are experts at formulating alternative treatments based on an individual's entire wellbeing and set-up. With a wide variety of remedies and tools at their disposal, the experts will ascertain the extent of the Lyme disease, the symptoms on display and the emotional and physical makeup of the victim. This unique approach means that no one Lyme disease solution is the same for all sufferers. After consultation with a trained homeopathic expert, a treatment plan involving the following remedies will be developed to give the greatest chance for success in any given situation:

- Arnica is very valuable in relieving muscle pain and soreness.

- Arsenicum Album helps alleviate extreme restlessness and burning joint pains.

- Carcinosin, Lac Canimum, and Thuja are beneficial for the symptoms associated with the disease.

- Gelsemium can be used to help treat fatigue and weakness.

- Mercurius is used for less common symptoms of Lyme disease such as sore throat, mouth ulcers, and excess salivation.

- Rhus Tox proves very effective in combating pain and stiffness.

- Sepia and Tellurium, when used in the initial stages of the disease, can help to halt the advancement of its symptoms.

Detoxing

The publicity that cleansing programs and diets has recently received outlines the importance of a body cleanse once in a while. In essence, a body cleanse rids the body of harmful toxins and washes the body of impurities. In addition, to offering the body a general clean, a cleanse can have a big effect on the body's ability to fight off Lyme disease.

Cleanses usually contain:

- Bowel and parasite cleanse;

- Dental cleanse (e.g., teeth cleaning);

- Kidney cleanse; and

- Liver and gallbladder cleanse.

As the market for cleanses and detox's becomes convoluted, it is important that anyone considering a body cleanse consults a qualified herbalist or naturopath. While all readily available cleanses are safe, the benefits that can be garnered from some outweigh others. Accordingly, the first cleanse is recommended to be conducted by a professional to fully customize the treatment and cleanse depending on the individual.

Fruits and Vegetables

In the same vein as our recommendation to keep a balanced diet and multi-vitamin plan, we also recommend the daily uptake of fruits to facilitate faster rates of healing and immunity. The Vitamin C present in citrus fruits, strawberries, peppers and can enrich a diet and work with the body's natural healing process to stave off the disease.

Cooling Down or Heating Up

When we're children we learn that most ailments and injuries can be treated with Ice. From our first sporting injury, to nasty falls in the playground cooling down the source of pain and inflammation has meant there's always been use for the frozen vegetables in the freezer. Because, Lyme disease is usually always associated with swelling and inflammation, the application of Ice can provide relief. Cycling the ice pack or bag (covered with a towel or hand cloth) on the affected area can dull the sensation caused by Lyme disease.

Castor Oil Heat Pack
In the same way, heat can also aid in controlling the pain and swelling cause by the tick bite and Lyme disease. Our recommended heating method involves the use of Castor Oil. Using the same method as the cooling technique, patients simply rub the castor oil on the affected area and apply heat. Heating pads are common in pharmacies as are hot water bottles and wheat bags, both of which act as decent substitutes.

Staying Hydrated

H20 is an essential requirement of the human body. The advice to drink up to three liters of water each day is sound. Water can aptly assist in the prevention of the formation of uric acid crystals, and help to eliminate the crystals once they have formed.

Our bodies need water in order to function properly. A well hydrated body is crucial in fighting off unwanted disease and the importance of water should not be underestimated when confronted with the symptoms of Lyme disease.

When added to the treatments offered by your doctor and the alternative efforts you intend to go to after reading this report, water is an easy (and free!) proactive step to take to improve the chances of an expeditious Lyme disease recovery.

The Institute of Medicine determined that an adequate intake (AI) for men is roughly 3 liters (about 13 cups) of total beverages a day.

The AI for women is 2.2 liters (about 9 cups) of total beverages a day.

Visualize

By this point you've probably broadened your view of treatment options for Lyme disease. Another option to add to that list, and again, it's under the guise of alternative treatments, is visualization. Research coming out of the Center for Nursing Research in New York proposes visualization as an alternative remedy but with a difference. In this treatment, you are instructed to visualize the very heart of the disease-the spirochete that causes Lyme disease. You are to imagine that you can see the spirochete swimming in your bloodstream, causing the damage to your body that you want to cure. Then, you imagine yourself, candle in hand, swimming in your own bloodstream. Reach out toward the spirochetes and watch them burn and die in the flame of your healing candle. Continue with the visualization until you picture your body free from the spirochetes and the disease altogether. The researchers suggest performing this visualization once a day, preferably in the morning, until healed.

While this may sound rather unorthodox, the results that some patients have encountered seem to suggest that it's worth the effort, especially if the psychological impact of Lyme disease is making you feel discouraged and disheartened.

This report offers a magnitude of treatment options, some may work for you and other mays not, but the important message to take out of the report is that there are options, and there are options that work for you.

Preventing Lyme Disease

Preventing Tick Bites

Having touched on the treatment options available, both in a traditional sense and in a holistic sense, it's also important to shed some light onto the ways in which to prevent the disease in the first place. As the quote goes "prevention is the best cure." Where ticks are ever present and the climate facilitates the breeding of ticks, it's crucial to take these preventative steps (especially in the coastal regions of the Northeast):

- Wear long sleeves and long pants tucked into your socks when performing outdoor activities.

- Consider wearing light-colored clothing so you are better able to see ticks if they are on you.

- Tie your hair back and wear a hat so that ticks cannot hide on you without you knowing it.

- When hiking along a trail, try to stay in the center of the path so that you do not brush up against hedges or overhanging brush and branches where ticks may be found.

- Spray your skin and clothing with appropriate insecticides to repel and/or kill ticks. Be careful, of course, to select the appropriate insecticides and be sure to read and follow the directions carefully.

- When coming in from outdoor activities, perform a "tick check" on yourself and all individuals who were exposed to the environment. Be sure to check behind the knees, between the fingers and toes, under the arms, in and behind the ears, and on the neck, hairline, and top of the head. Additionally, you'll want to examine those places on the body where your clothing presses on your bare skin. Ixode ticks are very small; look for a mark that resembles a small freckle or a piece of dirt.

- Shower after all outdoor activities. If a tick hasn't bitten you yet, it may simply wash off and go down the drain without causing any problems.

What Should You Do If You Find A Tick?

- If a tick is found, remove immediately with tweezers.

- Research indicates that it takes approximately 48 hours for an infected tick to transmit the Lyme bacterium.

- Remove the tick from the head, do not squeeze or handle the body.

- Save the tick on a piece of tape sealed in a plastic bag to confirm the identification.

- Swab the bite with an antiseptic.

- After outdoor outings, remove and wash clothing immediately.

To Remove a Tick:

- For best results, use fine-tipped tweezers to securely grasp the tick as close to your skin as possible.

- With equal grasp and a steady motion, pull the tick away from the location of the bite.

- Sometimes the tick's mouth parts will remain lodged in the skin. Don't panic; once the body has been removed, the tick can no longer transmit the disease. Over time, watch for signs of infection and soak the affected area in warm water to help remove any remaining body parts.

- Immediately clean the location with antibacterial soap and/or rubbing alcohol and warm water.

- Try not to crush the tick's body as this can transmit the disease and other bacteria. If you do crush it, wash your skin again with warm water, antibacterial soap and/or rubbing alcohol.

What Not to Do:

- Do not use a hot match, nail polish, or petroleum jelly to remove a tick. (These can actually have a detrimental effect on tick removal and cause the tick to burrow in, making extraction more difficult).

Pets and Lyme Disease

Notwithstanding the devastating impact Lyme disease can have on individuals, Lyme disease can also infect household pets with tragic consequences. The following chapter describes the preventative measures that you should take to keep your family pets free from ticks.

Lyme Disease Warning Signs

The difficulty is, that like humans, animals might show no symptoms of the disease. It is even trickier to pick up symptoms due to pets' inability to communicate their symptoms. This poses a worrying threat, as Lyme disease can cause eye, heart, kidney, and nervous system damage in animals if not treated. Having said that, here are some specific symptoms to look out for in your domestic pets.

Felines
Cats can show a variety of symptoms including: breathing issues, changes in appetite, eye problems, fatigue, fever, heart troubles, and lameness. However, many cats show no visible signs of infection.

Dogs
Dogs can show a variety of symptoms including: change of appetite, fevers and lethargy. Additionally, dogs can have arthritis-like pains, kidney and heart issues, and neurological complications. Indeed, dogs actually show many of the same symptoms that humans do.

Pet Lyme Disease Prevention

To help prevent Lyme disease in your pet, you'll want to do what you can to prevent your pets from being bitten by ticks. Follow these simple guidelines to keep your pets safe from ticks:

- Apply tick-killing chemicals to your pets; products (sprays and dips) containing permethrins and pyrethrins do a great job of killing ticks on dogs, and horses. Permethrins should NOT be used on cats.

- Place tick collars on your pets to keep ticks from biting.

- Apply specific insecticides to your yard that kill ticks.

- Be smart about where you let your pets roam. Keep your grass cut short to keep the tick population down.

- Make sure you check your pets for ticks on a regular basis, especially after they have been exposed to areas that have a greater chance for tick habitation.

- If you find a tick, remove it in the same way you would for a human. Be sure watch your pet in the days that follow to see if the pet displays any signs of infection. If you notice any abnormalities, see your vet immediately.

Final Thoughts

This report has given an overview of Lyme disease, the possible treatment plans to handle the disease, and the preventative measures that can be taken to prevent the possibility of an initial infection. With particular emphasis on holistic therapies and alternative treatments, we've explained the benefits in great detail of supplementing traditional medicinal measures with a balanced diet, multi-vitamins, herbs and cleanses. The seventy two hour cleanse and home remedy kit supports of our research findings and can help victims of the nasty tick disease rid themselves of infection and alleviate their suffering within the aforementioned seventy two hours.

We believe our report will further educate the population on the risks associated with Lyme disease to people and household pets, but we also hope that it provides the light at the end of the tunnel for those that are struggling with their strain of the disease and their unique symptoms. Our system of overall health, combined with our innovative ways to naturally manage and treat your Lyme disease, are entirely safe and should hold you in good stead for combatting your illness and improving your general health and reaction to further infections and ailments.

Thank you for taking the time to educate yourself on Lyme disease and for reading our report. We hope that the information is useful and informative and as always we wish you well on your journey toward good health!

Newsletter Special Offer

Visit and sign up for Nature's Natural Health newsletter to get health and wellness tips delivered to your email.

www.naturesnaturalhealth.com/join/